How do we manage:

ACNE

How do we manage:

ACNE

Thomas Francis Poyner
MB BS MRCP MRCGP DRCOG DPD

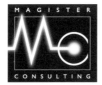

MAGISTER CONSULTING LTD

Published in the UK by
Magister Consulting Ltd
The Old Rectory
St Mary's Way
Stone
Dartford
Kent BR3 5LE
UK

Copyright © 1999 Magister Consulting Ltd

Printed and bound in Great Britain by Bishops Printers Ltd.

ISBN 1 873839 56 1

Acknowledgements

To Robin, Beth and all those loveable teenagers with spots.

Contents

Chapter One

Understanding Acne   1

   Introduction   1

   Acne – a common problem   1

   Natural history of acne   2

   Pathophysiology   2

   Acne and drugs   4

   Acne and the environment   4

Chapter Two

Is it Acne?   7

   The rash of acne   7

   The diagnosis of acne   9

   Conditions associated with acne   9

   The differential diagnosis of acne   9

   Complications of acne   13

Chapter Three

How Patients Present   15

   Consultations in primary care   15

   Referrals to secondary care   16

   Grading the patient's acne   17

   Psychological aspects of acne   18

Chapter Four

Treating Acne   25

   Aims of treatment   25

   The cost of acne   26

Chapter Five

Topical Treatments for Acne   27

    Benzoyl peroxide   28

    Azelaic acid   28

    Topical antibiotics   28

    Topical retinoids   29

    Nicotinamide   30

    Salicylic acid   31

    Sulphur   31

    Using a combination of topical treatments   31

Chapter Six

Systemic Therapies   33

    Oral antibiotics   33

    Antibiotic resistance   37

    Combined oral and topical therapy   38

Chapter Seven

The Female Patient   41

    The female with acne   41

    Hormones and hormonal therapy   41

    Interactions   44

    Erythromycin as first choice?   44

    The pregnant female   44

Chapter Eight

Oral Retinoids   47

    Indications for oral retinoids   47

    The dosage of isotretinoin   48

    Outcome of retinoids   49

Advice to patients on oral retinoids   49

Local side-effects of retinoids   49

Possible laboratory abnormalities and screening
  with oral retinoids   49

Systemic side-effects   50

Teratogenicity   50

Repeated courses of isotretinoin   50

Chapter Nine

Protocol for Treating Acne in Primary Care   51

  Mild acne   51

  Moderate acne   52

  Topical agents   54

  Oral antibiotics   55

  Review   55

  Severe acne   56

Chapter Ten

Audit of Acne   57

Chapter Eleven

Physical Steps in Acne Treatment   59

  Cryotherapy   59

  Injection of cysts   60

  Phototherapy   60

  Treatment of scarring   60

  Treatment of comedones   61

  Unusual systemic therapies   61

Appendix I

Self-help   63

Appendix II

Formulary   65

    Systemic Treatment   65

    Topical Drugs   66

    Topical Antimicrobial Drugs   67

    Topical Antibiotics   68

    Topical Retinoids   69

References   71

Index   77

Chapter One

Understanding acne

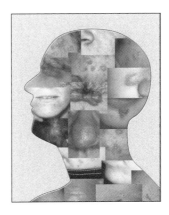

Introduction

Acne is a very common problem, affecting visible sites and causing physiological and psychological scarring for many people
(Figure 1). There is no mystery to acne; the diagnosis is easily
made and most treatments can be instituted in primary care.
General practitioners would be able to treat more patients and
make fewer referrals if they received ongoing education in dermatology, especially on acne[1].

Acne – a common problem

Virtually everyone has acne at some time in their lives, although
for most people it is minor. We do know that 2% of the population
consult doctors for diseases of the sebaceous glands[2]. The prevalence of moderate to severe acne in one study was approximately
14% in those between 15 and 24 years of age[3].

A few patients develop infantile acne (Figure 2), which is thought to be due to maternal androgens. For the vast majority acne starts around puberty and gradually deteriorates thereafter. There is no difference in incidence between the sexes. Females, having an earlier puberty than males, may develop acne at a younger age, however the androgen drive in the teens can result in males having more severe acne. Moderate and severe acne has been found to be more common in males in a senior high school[4]. There is a genetic link to acne, and a positive family history may be elicited in those with severe acne. Some races have less acne than others. The prevalence of severe acne is possibly in decline, affecting 0.6–1.4% of young adults. There has been a shift in severity to more milder cases.

Natural history of acne

Without treatment, acne remains static for a few years, then for many it gradually improves in the mid-twenties. However, for some, the rash continues. Facial acne is more common in adult women than men, with an estimated prevalence of 11%[5]. Acne is becoming a problem for a significant number of patients in middle age. By the age of 40, 5% of women and 1% of men have a problem[6].

Two main clinical groups with post-adolescent acne have been identified. There are those with persistent acne and those with late-onset acne. A minority of women also have features of hyper-androgenicity.

Pathophysiology

Acne is a disease of the sebaceous glands and occurs at most sites, with the greatest density on the face, chest and back. The only sites not to have sebaceous glands are the palms of the hands and the soles of the feet. The glands need androgens to stimulate the production of sebum, and there is a physiological increase in androgens at puberty. The sensitivity of the receptors of the pilosebaceous follicle is thought to be more important than any endocrine abnormality. When tested, males with acne have normal levels of androgens. Patients with virilizing tumours can develop acne (although these tumours are rare) and have other signs of abnormal hormone production.

There is a laboratory-detectable hormonal abnormality in up to half of the females with acne. They may have slightly higher levels of free testosterone, but this does not need treatment. There is an association between acne and polycystic ovaries, and minor degrees of this syndrome have been revealed with the improvements in ultrasound.

The enzyme '5-alpha reductase' is involved in the conversion of testosterone to its more potent metabolite dihydrotestosterone. This enzyme is thought to play some part in the development of acne and androgenetic alopecia.

In acne there is hyperproliferation of the cells lining the ducts of the pilosebaceous follicle. These cells adhere to the duct walls and produce partial obstruction. The hyperconification is under the control of androgens and leads to the formation of the microcomedones. Closed lesions are known as whiteheads and open lesions blackheads. The colour of blackheads is due to pigment. Comedones are initial acne lesions.

Secondarily, the obstructed ducts may become colonized by bacteria. These include *Propionibacterium* acnes, *Staphylococcus epidermidis* and *Pityrosporum ovale*. The *Propionibacterium* acnes have the ability to break down triglycerides in sebum to free fatty acids by producing a lipase. The bacterial colonization is associated with the release of inflammatory mediators such as cytokines. There is a polymorph and lymphocyte infiltrate in acne, and there may be pus formation. The ducts may eventually rupture, which contributes to the development of large inflammatory lesions.

Acne and drugs

Those self-medicating with anabolic steroids may develop acne, but this resolves on cessation of the anabolic steroids. Prescribed oral, topical and rarely inhaled steroids may cause or exacerbate acne. Acne is also associated with the taking of anticonvulsants and lithium.

Acne and the environment

Holidays in sunny destinations are usually beneficial, although some patients relapse because of high humidity. The condition known as 'Acne Majorca' is due to the combined effects of the humid environment and oily sunscreens. Working in hot, humid environments can also be deleterious. Simply, if you suffer with acne, keep out of the kitchen and the tropics! Cosmetics can make acne worse, and patients who want to use cosmetics should use light, water-based ones. Working with aromatic hydrocarbons, coal tar and cutting oils can also cause acne.

Acne can be induced by physical means. Violinists may develop it under their chins: the so-called 'fiddler's neck'. Constant rubbing of clothing on the neck with, for example, turtle- or polo-neck sweaters can result in acne. Diet is not a factor in the causation of acne. Smoking may have a beneficial effect, possibly due to an anti-inflammatory effect from nicotine, however this habit is not to be condoned[7]. Halogenated hydrocarbons and cutting oils can make acne worse, and there are reports of acne after use of a cow udder ointment[8].

Chapter Two

Is it acne?

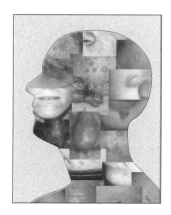

The rash of acne

Acne occurs at sites where follicles with sebaceous glands are plentiful. It does not affect the scalp because the scalp hair seems to have a protective effect. When examining acne, check all possible affected sites. The severity at one site can be quite different at another. Do not presume that the back is not significantly affected just because the acne is mild on the face. Examine the various lesions which can be present and look for scarring (Figure 3).

In acne there are non-inflamed lesions of open and closed comedones. The inflamed lesions include papules, pustules, cysts and nodules.

Comedones

Non-inflamed lesions are known as blackheads and whiteheads (Figure 4). Open comedones (blackheads) are produced by hyperkeratinization of the follicular duct. The dark colour is due to melanin. Obstruction of the duct produces closed comedones (whiteheads) with distended pilosebaceous follicles. Comedones are initial acne elements.

Inflamed lesions

Some comedones resolve whilst others persist. Comedones, especially the closed ones, go on to become inflamed lesions, although some inflamed lesions develop *de novo*. These inflamed lesions are either superficial or deep, and superficial ones are known as papules. Such lesions are raised and red and may progress to pustules (Figure 5), which may discharge. Most superficial papules and pustules last between 1 and 2 weeks. Some pustules are deeper and take longer to resolve (Figure 6). Nodules and cysts are deep inflamed lesions which can be painful. They last between 2 and 8 weeks, and are associated with scarring.

Macules

Macules are the end result of resolving inflamed lesions. They last for weeks before resolving and some lesions result in atrophic macules.

Scars

Approximately 17% of patients develop scarring. Scarring may develop with any grade of acne, with deep inflammatory lesions, although it is more common in those whose acne is more severe, some patients are more prone to scarring. Scarring may result either in a loss or an increase in tissue. Loss of tissue can produce superficial soft scars, depressed fibrotic scars, and ice-pick scars. An increase in collagen results in hypertrophic and keloid scars, which are raised and linear, often found on the shoulders (Figure 7).

The diagnosis of acne

There is usually little difficulty in making the diagnosis of acne. View the face, chest and back, as the severity can be disproportionate between these sites. It is important to make the examination with good lighting and to palpate lesions. To make the diagnosis, look for the classical acne lesions of open and closed comedones, papules and pustules (Figures 8 and 9). Rosacea may have a similar appearance, but there are no comedones. Healing acne lesions can go through a macular stage, and this can cause confusion with macules which have become atrophic scars.

Conditions associated with acne

Hidradenitis suppurativa

This is a chronic inflammatory disease of apocrine glands. It is found in the flexures, affecting the axillae, groin and perineum. *Hidradenitis suppurativa* (Figure 10) can coexist with acne, and there are a lot of similarities between the two conditions. The rash presents with papules, pustules, nodules, abscesses and sinuses, and there may be scarring. It can be treated medically with oral antibiotics and antiandrogens, but some cases require surgery.

The differential diagnosis of acne

Rosacea

This is the most common differential diagnosis. Rosacea (Figure 11) is a chronic inflammatory facial skin condition of unknown cause. One theory suggests that it may represent long-term photodamage, and another is that it is a vascular disorder. The *Demodex* mite has been implicated in the natural history of this condition. Its age of onset is usually later than that of acne. More females are affected than males, though the latter tend to be more severely affected, and the disease is more common in fair-skinned Celts. Facial erythema occurs in a cruciate distribution, with flushing. There are papules and pustules but no comedones. Rosacea may be associated with blepharitis and conjunctivitis, and the nose can become thickened, producing a bulbous and irregular swelling known as a rhinophyma (Figure 12).

As regards treatment, rosacea responds to oral tetracyclines and topical metronidazole. If facial flushing is a major problem, oral clonidine may be beneficial. Severe cases of rosacea (Figure 13) can be treated with oral retinoids. Laser treatment may be used for facial telangiectasia, whilst surgery may be appropriate to treat a rhinophyma.

Acne agminata

This rash is of unknown aetiology and tends to affect young adults, who develop yellowish–brown papules on the face. Such lesions resolve in 1–2 years, leaving scars.

Acne necrotica

This condition affects adult males and presents as itchy, painful papules and pustules. The papules undergo necrosis and leave scars.

Acne keloid

This is a chronic inflammatory condition in which pustules develop in the nape of the neck and eventually scar.

Comedo naevus

These can develop on the face, scalp and trunk, and lesions can be present at birth or develop later. There are comedones and occasionally inflammatory lesions.

Epidermoid cysts

These have a punctum, presenting as cheesy material (Figure 14). The cysts may become infected and inflamed. Boils due to a staphylococcal infection may develop on the face.

Milia

Milia are small, white cysts, and a common site is on the eyelid. They differ from the lesions of acne in the lack of a punctum and they can be pricked with a sterile needle.

Perioral dermatitis

Young females may develop papules and pustules around the mouth, which may result from the inappropriate use of topical steroids. Perioral dermatitis (Figure 15) responds to a course of oral antibiotics and withdrawal of topical steroids.

Pityrosporum folliculitis

This condition is found on teenagers and young adults, and is associated with exposure to sun. It presents as multiple tiny, itchy papules and pustules on the shoulders and back. There are no comedones, and the condition responds to topical imidazoles.

Seborrhoeic dermatitis

This is a scaly erythematous rash which can occur on the face, chest (figure 16) and scalp. The rash frequently affects the nasolabial folds and ears. The chest is red and scaly, and the scale is rather greasy (Figure 16). Petaloid lesions may be found over the sternum.

Senile comedones

These occur when debris accumulates in the pilosebaceous duct, and are often associated with ageing (Figure 17). The appearance of senile comedones can simulate a basal cell carcinoma. However, the contents are easily expressed, making the diagnosis clear.

Steatocystoma multiplex

This condition is rare and may be inherited. Patients develop multiple cysts which can become inflamed.

Sycosis barbae

Sycosis barbae is an infection of the beard area with *Staphylococcus aureus*. Treatments include appropriate oral antibiotics and topical antiseptics. *Pseudo-sycosis barbae* is found in Afro-Caribbean males, and is due to curly hairs growing back into the skin of the beard area.

Tinea barbae

This is due to a dermatophyte infection of the beard area. The fungal infection is transmitted from animals; it therefore commonly affects farm workers. The rash is quite aggressive with inflammation and pustules. Samples should be taken for mycological examination.

Tuberous sclerosis

Patients with this rare, inherited condition can present with papules on the face, especially around the nose, known as adenoma sebaceum. They can have hyperplastic gums and 'Shagreen patches' (found on the lower back, these are connective tissue naevi and appear as yellow plaques with a cobblestone surface). Visual problems are common, along with epilepsy and mental retardation.

Complications of acne

Gram-negative folliculitis

This condition can occur during treatment of acne with antibiotics. There is often a flare of acne with multiple pustules. It is worth taking a swab, discontinuing treatment with the current antibiotic, and then treating with appropriate antibiotics. Proteus is a common pathogen. The pathogens can be cultured from the patient's nose, and amoxycillin or trimethoprim are often suitable antibiotic treatments. A Gram-negative folliculitis can also be treated with an oral retinoid.

Post-inflammatory hyperpigmentation

Post-inflammatory hyperpigmentation can be a problem, especially for Afro-Caribbean patients. This condition may take a couple of years to resolve, but treatment can be attempted with topical azelaic acid, although prevention is best if early effective acne treatment is used.

Acne excoriee

Acne excoriee is found in young females. It results from repeated picking, and in many ways resembles prurigo. Caring for the psyche is as important as treatment of the acne.

Pyoderma faciale

This condition is rare, and only affects females. Patients often have mild to moderate acne and under certain circumstances go on to develop a sudden flare of their acne. Stress may be a factor. Patients develop multiple pustular lesions, but despite this remain well, unlike those with acne fulminans.

Acne conglobata

This severe form of acne presents with large nodules, abscesses and sinuses. It is more common in males and those living in tropical climates. There is suppuration and scarring, and the condition may be associated with *hidradenitis suppurativa*. Patients can be successfully treated with oral retinoids.

Acne fulminans

In this form of acne there is an immune reaction to the *Propionibacterium* acnes. Classically, it affects male patients who have truncal nodular acne. Patients develop a fever, malaise, and frequently a polyarthropathy, and have a vasculitis and possibly an erythema nodosum. The general systemic upset is accompanied by a leucocytosis, and there may be a painful spleen. Treatment is with high-dose steroids and oral antibiotics.

Chapter Three

How patients present

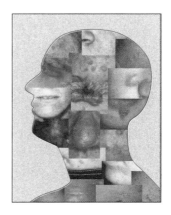

Consultations in primary care

The majority of teenagers develop acne, although only 15% consult. There can be a delay of 3–4 years before patients seek help from their GP. Reducing the delay in initiating treatment would reduce the risk of scarring, but many teenagers do not feel that their GP will be interested and therefore delay consulting. Explain to the teenager the cause of acne, and that it is a treatable condition. Ascertain the sites and severity of the acne, and record any scarring and psychological problems.

When patients were asked with whom they could discuss openly their acne problems, the GP scored highly (72%) compared to the dermatologist (50%) and pharmacist (6%)[9].

It is important to involve the practice team in treating acne. Patients often find the practice nurse less threatening than the GP.

The practice nurse is able to advise on acne and its treatment and can also provide the follow-up for many patients on treatment. During such consultations there are opportunities to provide advice on problems associated with acne therapies, such as interactions between oral antibiotics and oral contraceptives. Health visitors can liaise with schools to provide health education on topics such as acne. This enables those who may develop acne to be targeted with health education.

Involvement of the community pharmacist can lead to a common policy on acne treatment. This enables more patients to be treated without an undue drain on the practice's time and budget. The pharmacist can provide advice and appropriate 'over-the-counter' medication for those with mild acne, whilst patients receiving prescriptions may receive advice from the pharmacist on the appropriate use of medication.

The psychological problems experienced by the patient do not always correlate with the severity of the acne, so inquiry should be made into psychological well-being. When patients consult it is important to dispel myths. Diet has no part in the causation of acne; furthermore, there is no correlation between lack of hygiene and acne.

Advise the patient on the speed of action of medication, as this will aid compliance. There is seldom a response from oral antibiotics before 6 weeks. A 50% improvement in 3 months is desirable, although the response is often slower, and there should be a review every 2–3 months.

Referrals to secondary care

Most treatments for acne can be delivered in primary care. Secondary care is expensive and rather impersonal. Referral of those with mild to moderate acne who have not received appropriate treatment is a waste of valuable resources.

Approximately 15% of patients with significant acne are referred to a dermatologist. Those with severe nodulocystic acne need urgent referral. However, there should be no delay in instituting initial therapy. Patients with moderate to severe acne which is unresponsive to adequate therapy need referral. Approximately 5% of patients do not respond to conventional therapy, such as an oral antibiotic combined with an appropriate topical therapy. Patients whose acne relapses repetitively after three consecutive courses of treatment should be referred. Patients with scarring, despite treatment, need referral. Patients with dysmorphophobia (a body image disorder) form a problematical group which benefits from specialist care.

Contents of the referral letter

The referral letter should state clearly what the GP and patient hope to achieve from the referral. Any background information is helpful, i.e. the types of therapies used and their dosage and duration. For female patients it is essential to know what contraceptive advice has been given. Issues concerning likely compliance need airing. If the referral is made with a recommendation to use oral retinoids, then it is very helpful if the GP has performed initial laboratory screening, including tests on liver function, blood sugar and fasting lipids.

Grading the patient's acne

It is important to be able to grade acne; it enables the most appropriate therapy to be prescribed and progress to be monitored at follow-up. Dermatology departments have complex grading systems, and this tends to deter GPs. In general practice, acne is recorded simply as mild, moderate or severe. Look for scarring and record any psychological aspects.

View the acne in a good light and remember to palpate lesions. It is important to examine all possible sites. Almost all patients have facial involvement, and many also on the chest and back. Record the severity at different sites. Acne on the back is often quite resistant to treatment, and topical treatments are often difficult to apply. Record any scarring. Table 1 shows a simple method of grading acne.

Table 1 – A simple method of grading acne

Type of acne	Findings
Mild	Comedones
	A few small papules
	A few pustules
Moderate	Numerous comedones and small
	inflammatory papules
	Numerous pustules
Severe	Numerous comedones, deeper papules
	and pustules. Deep and larger leisions
	Presence of cysts and absesses

Psychological aspects of acne

Acne has a major impact on patients' lives. It involves a visible site which makes it difficult to hide. At puberty, appearance and body image take on major roles. Acne therefore causes embarrassment and makes people feel unattractive. Some individuals have reduced self-confidence and others go on to develop a distorted body image. Acne may lead to underachievement at school and reduce the patient's chances of entering employment. Acne can interfere with sporting activities because the patient may not want to expose his/her body to team-mates in changing rooms.

The risk of suicide associated with dermatological conditions has been highlighted in one study which reported 16 deaths (seven men and nine women) of patients who had presented to two dermatologists. Most of the patients had either dysmorphophobia or acne[10].

Measures of disability

It is useful to measure the disability resulting from diseases, and there are general health questionnaires such as the 'Sickness Impact Profile' and the 'SF-36' which attempt to do this. There are specific questionnaires concerning dermatology, such as the 'Dermatology Life Quality Index' (DLQI) and the 'Children's Dermatology Life Quality Index' (CDLQI). There is also a wide range of disease-specific questionnaires. The Department of Dermatology in Cardiff developed initially an acne disability index[11], which has now been superseded by the 'Cardiff Acne Disability Index' (CADI), which is the most suitable routine measurement in primary care. The 'Assessments of the Psychological and Social Effects of Acne' (APSEA) has also been developed in Leeds.

Cardiff Acne Disability Index (CADI)

1. As a result of acne, during the last month have you been aggressive, frustrated or embarrassed?

   a) *Very much indeed*

   b) *A lot*

   c) *A little*

   d) *Not at all*

2. Do you think that having acne during the last month interfered with your daily social life, social events or relationships with members of the opposite sex?

   a) *Severely, affecting all activities*

   b) *Moderate, in most activities*

   c) *Occasionally or in only some activities*

   d) *Not at all*

3. During the last month have you avoided public changing facilities or wearing costumes because of your acne?

   a) *All the time*

   b) *Most of the time*

   c) *Occasionally*

   d) *Not at all*

4. How would you describe your feelings about the appearance of your skin over the last month?

   a) *Very depressed and miserable*

   b) *Usually concerned*

   c) *Occasionally concerned*

   d) *Not bothered*

5. Please indicate how bad you think your acne is now:

   a) *The worst it could possibly be*

   b) *A major problem*

   c) *A minor problem*

   d) *Not a problem*

Each question is scored 0–3 (d=0, c=1, b=2 and a=3). To ascertain the degree of disability the score from the five answers is added up to give the final score within a range of 0–15.

Reproduced by kind permission of Dr RJ Motley and Dr AY Finlay[12]

The APSEA was designed to be used as a quick and effective means of assessing the psychopathological effects of acne. It correlates well with other indices and is especially sensitive in assessing acne scarring.

Assessments of the Psychological and Social Effects Of Acne (APSEA)

In numbers 1–6 tick the most appropriate answer to each question.

In the last week

1. Worrying thoughts through my mind
   A great deal of the time
   A lot of the time
   From time to time, not often
   Only occasionally

2. I sit at ease and feel relaxed
   Definitely
   Usually
   Not often
   Not at all

3. I feel restless, as if I have to be on the move
   Very much indeed
   Quite a lot
   Not very much
   Not at all

At this moment

4. I like what I look like in photographs
   Not at all
   Sometimes
   Very often
   Nearly all the time

5. I wished I looked better
   Not at all
   Sometimes
   Very often
   Nearly all the time

6. On the whole I am satisfied with myself
   Strongly disagree
   Disagree
   Agree
   Strongly agree

In numbers 7–15 read the following carefully and put a line at the point that most accurately represents how you feel.

7. I still enjoy the things I used to
   Never   0   1   2   3   4   5   6   7   8   9   10   All the time

8. I am more irritable than usual
   Never   0   1   2   3   4   5   6   7   8   9   10   All the time

9. I feel that I am useful and needed
   Never   0   1   2   3   4   5   6   7   8   9   10   All the time

How has your skin condition limited the following activities or made them more difficult or awkward, or less enjoyable since you have had acne?

10. Going shopping
    Not at all   0   1   2   3   4   5   6   7   8   9   10   All the time

11. Going out socially to meet friends from outside the home
    Not at all   0   1   2   3   4   5   6   7   8   9   10   All the time

12. Going away for weekends, holidays and outings

Not at all 0 1 2 3 4 5 6 7 8 9 10 *All the time*

13. Eating out

Not at all 0 1 2 3 4 5 6 7 8 9 10 *All the time*

14. Using public changing rooms/swimming pools

Not at all 0 1 2 3 4 5 6 7 8 9 10 *All the time*

15. Do you think your appearance will interfere with your chances of future employment?

Strongly   *Strongly*

disagree 0 1 2 3 4 5 6 7 8 9 10 *agree*

Questions 1–6 are scored from 0–9, and questions 10–15 are scored from 0–10. The highest score is 144, and patients with a high APSEA score would benefit from early effective treatment.

Reproduced by kind permission of Dr AM Layton and Professor WJ Cunliffe[13]

Chapter Four

Treating acne

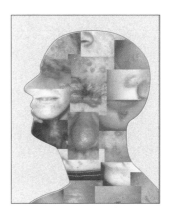

Aims of treatment

The aims of treatment should be to improve the patient's acne and prevent scarring. Improvement in the rash helps the patient's psychological well-being. Scarring is very difficult to treat, and prevention is better than cure. Appropriate treatment can prevent scarring, and delay in initial treatment can lead to scarring.

Appropriate therapy depends on the site, type and severity of the acne. Topical therapies are ideal for mild to moderate acne, and combined topical and oral therapies should be used for moderate to severe acne. Those with severe acne need dermatological referral, but this should not be an excuse for not initiating therapy. To treat acne consistently one needs to perform a simple grading exercise, assess any psychological factors, and then use a protocol. It is important to involve the patient when deciding the most appropriate therapy. Some patients may prefer to use a topical therapy, whilst others prefer systemic therapy. The site of the acne (in particular on the back) sometimes makes the use of topical treatments difficult.

Teenagers often have unreasonable expectations of the speed of action of treatments: they want their spots 'gone by tomorrow'. This expectation leads to disillusionment and poor compliance. Education of patients can counteract these negative factors, but information needs to be tailored to the patient, taking into account their age and intelligence. Future teenagers will no doubt surf the Internet to become informed about their acne; this may further challenge a GP's knowledge of the possible therapies available.

The cost of acne

It is important to take note of the cost of prescribing for acne. In 1992, there were 3.5 million consultations for acne, resulting in 51,000 dermatological referrals. The cost of a dermatology referral is approximately £60. It has been estimated that acne prescribing accounts for approximately £44.8 million a year of the NHS budget.

The cost-effectiveness of a particular medication is frequently highlighted. A GP has to decide what should be first-line therapy, second-line therapy, and what should be held in reserve. Such decisions are often taken either in a practice or by using local guidelines. One can look at the costs in different ways; the cost per drug, per prescription, per month of treatment, or the total cost of treating a patient are relevant. A drug such as oral isotretinoin may appear expensive, but undue delay in prescribing it can result in repeated courses of oral antibiotic, as well as the cost of a course of oral retinoids.

Chapter Five

Topical treatments for acne

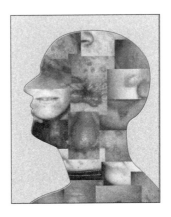

Topical therapies are suitable for treating those with mild to moderate acne. Many systemic therapies benefit from being taken alongside the application of a topical therapy. A whole range of topical therapies for acne are available. These therapies act in different ways. Unlike systemic therapies, topical therapies do not have the disadvantages of systemic side-effects and interactions. Topical therapies include:

- Benzoyl peroxide
- Nicotinamide
- Topical retinoids
- Sodium sulfacetamide

- Azelaic acid
- Topical antibiotics
- Salicylic acid
- Sulphur

Benzoyl peroxide

Benzoyl peroxide has been available for many years and is a well-tested treatment, becoming the 'gold standard' of topical therapies. It has antibacterial and some keratolytic activity. It is an oxidizing agent, so unlike antibiotics, bacterial resistance cannot develop. Irritation is the most common problem with benzoyl peroxide treatment. Occasionally, patients develop a contact allergic dermatitis. Benzoyl peroxide can cause bleaching of hair, clothes and bedding.

Benzoyl peroxide is available as a 2.5%, 5% or 10% concentration. The problem of irritation may reduce compliance and acceptability, but can be overcome by applying emollients to reduce the dryness of the skin, or by applying a topical steroid short-term. Patients should begin by applying the 2.5% strength once-daily, and then gradually increase the area treated and the frequency of application to twice-daily. If patients can tolerate the 2.5% strength, the dose can be increased to the 5% strength, although only a few patients are able to tolerate the 10% concentration.

Azelaic acid

Azelaic acid has some antibacterial, anticomedonal and anti-inflammatory properties. It may normalize the follicular keratinization. Its main advantage is in being less irritant than benzoyl peroxide. Azelaic acid has roughly the same clinical effect as benzoyl peroxide, but causes less irritation. It is available as a 20% cream, applied once-daily for 1 week, then twice-daily for up to 6 months. Azelaic acid rarely causes photosensitivity, and should not be used during pregnancy or lactation. Azelaic acid can be used to treat post-inflammatory pigmentation.

Topical antibiotics

Topical antibiotics have a direct antibacterial and anti-inflammatory effect. They have little or no anticomedonal activity. They have the advantage of causing little irritation, and are effective at tackling any premenstrual flare. Topical antibiotics should be effective and have no resistance. Ideally, topical antibiotics should not be used systemically. Chloramphenicol and neomycin have been used as topical therapies, but can cause sensitization.

Tetracycline, which is frequently taken orally to treat acne, was one of the earliest antibiotics to be used topically. It can produce fluorescence under UV light, which can be a problem in discos.

Topical clindamycin is both an effective and acceptable treatment for acne. It is applied twice-daily, either as a 1% solution in an alcohol base or as a lotion in an aqueous base. The aqueous formulation is effective if there are excoriated areas (Figure 18).

Topical clindamycin reduces *Propionibacterium* acnes more effectively than topical erythromycin in vivo, but clinical trials indicate that their efficacy is similar. Erythromycin is a popular treatment for acne because it has a wide safety margin. However, bacterial resistance to erythromycin and clindamycin is an increasing problem. The addition of zinc or benzoyl peroxide to topical erythromycin may overcome bacterial resistance and also help the penetration of the erythromycin.

Topical retinoids

Topical retinoids are anticomedogenic. They reverse the abnormality of hyperconification in the pilosebaceous duct and stop the formation of microcomedones. Therefore they are very useful in treating acne as they unblock the pores. Topical retinoids are used in primary care to treat acne and psoriasis. Recently, they have also been shown to have an effect on solar damage. Topical retinoids may cause irritation, which can result in redness and peeling. This can be reduced by using an emollient or spacing the applications. Topical retinoids may cause photosensitization, although restriction to evening use only overcomes this problem. Therefore care has to be taken if the medication is applied during the daytime. Oral retinoids are teratogenic, so patients are advised not to use topical retinoids in pregnancy.

Topical tretinoin and isotretinoin

Topical retinoids include tretinoin and its isomer, isotretinoin. Tretinoin is available as a gel, lotion and cream formulation. The cream and lotion are formulated as a 0.025% concentration, whereas the gel has two strengths: 0.01% and 0.025%. Isotretinoin is available as a gel (0.05%), and can be used once- or twice-daily.

Adapalene

Adapalene is a topical retinoid receptor agonist used for the treatment of acne. It possesses some of the properties of topical retinoids, but has a low potential for irritation. It has comedolytic activity and an anti-inflammatory action, and is suitable for mild to moderate acne. It is applied as an aqueous gel, once-daily before retiring. Adapalene gel 0.1% was shown in a large clinical study to provide superior efficacy and better tolerability than tretinoin gel 0.025%[14]. Adapalene 0.1% cream formulation is also on the market for patients with more sensitive dry skin. Adapalene-like topical retinoids should not to be used during pregnancy or lactation.

Nicotinamide

Nicotinamide is an effective treatment for mild to moderate acne. It acts against inflammatory lesions by interfering with inflammatory mediators and inhibiting neutrophil activity. It is available as a 4% gel which is applied twice-daily. Dryness and irritation of the skin may result.

Salicylic acid

Salicylic acid is a rather irritating keratolytic agent. A 2% solution is used as an acne treatment, although it has been superseded by topical retinoids.

Sulphur

This is a very old remedy and may have been used as a scabicide by the Egyptians. It is still used in combination with salicylic acid to treat seborrhoeic eczema and was previously used as an acne treatment with the intention of inducing desquamation. However, it is now only of historical interest.

Using a combination of topical treatments

It is logical to use a combination of topical therapies. Topical retinoids act especially against comedones, whilst topical antibiotics and benzoyl peroxide treat inflammatory lesions and reduce *Propionibacterium* acnes. Because they work in different ways, and are specific for different components of the disease, their benefits in combination are at least additive. It is also possible to minimize the likelihood of bacterial resistance by using combination therapy. Initial attempts at using dual therapy involved the use of one preparation in the morning and another in the evening. Combining the therapy usually improves compliance, and may in some cases reduce the irritation of one component. Benzoyl peroxide is available in combination with erythromycin, which should reduce the likelihood of resistance of *Propionibacterium* acnes. A product containing erythromycin combined with zinc is also available, which again reduces bacterial resistance.

A combination product of a topical retinoid (isotretinoin 0.05%) with topical erythromycin (2%) is available as a gel, which is applied once- or twice-daily. Similar advice is required when prescribing a topical retinoid.

A manufactured cream containing miconazole (2%) in combination with benzoyl peroxide (5%) is also available. Imidazoles, whilst not a first-line treatment, do have antibacterial and antifungal properties which can be effective, especially when the patient has dual pathologies.

Chapter Six

Systemic therapies

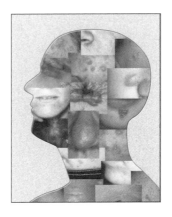

Oral antibiotics

Oral antibiotics are the standard therapy for moderate and moderate to severe acne. They are also the most appropriate therapy whilst severe acne patients are awaiting hospital appointments. Oral antibiotic therapies include oxytetracycline, doxycycline, lymecycline, minocycline and erythromycin. These antibiotics are active against *Propionibacterium* acnes and also have a direct anti-inflammatory effect. Their usage may be limited by side-effects, and may cause gastrointestinal upsets. Oral antibiotics may interact with other medications, including oral contraceptives and anticoagulants.

Tetracyclines should not be given to patients with renal failure. Females on tetracyclines can develop a candidal vulvovaginitis, and patients occasionally develop phototoxicity. A fixed drug eruption has been reported with tetracycline. Benign raised intracranial pressure is even rarer, although the possibility of this side-effect is increased if tetracyclines are taken with oral retinoids. Tetracyclines can be deposited in teeth and bones, and must not be prescribed to pregnant females, those who are breastfeeding, and children under 12 years of age.

Dosage of common oral antibiotics

The usual recommended dose of oxytetracycline or erythromycin is 500 mg twice-daily. Previously, the suggested initial dosage was 250 mg twice-daily, although the higher dosage is more effective. It has been recently suggested that the dosage should be 250 mg four times daily, because the half-life of these antibiotics is only 6 hours[15]. Whether the four times a day dosage or the twice-daily dosage regime is clinically important is not yet proven. After 3 months therapy of 1 g daily, the dose may be reduced if the desired clinical effect is obtained. Doxycycline, lymecycline and minocycline are recommended with one capsule per day dosage which is very convenient for patients and improves compliance. They can also be taken with food or milk and their absorption is not modified. The maximum improvement should be expected after 4–6 months, although some patients need longer courses. Certainly, males with truncal acne tend to be slower responders. Tetracycline and erythromycin need to be taken on an empty stomach as absorption is reduced by food, although some patients have difficulty in complying.

Oxytetracycline

Oxytetracyline is a good first-line treatment for acne. The absorption of oxytetracycline is reduced by concurrent administration of iron, calcium and antacids. Dairy products may also reduce its absorption. Oxytetracycline should be taken 30 minutes before food intake, and 4 hours after the last meal.

Erythromycin

Erythromycin is widely used for skin and soft tissue infections. However, there is an associated risk of developing increased bacterial resistance. Many therefore suggest that tetracycline should be the first-line antibiotic. Erythromycin does have some advantages, especially its use in pregnancy. It should not be used in those with liver disease. Erythromycin can interact with a number of medications, including terfenadine, astemizole, carbamazepine, cisapride and cyclosporin.

Doxycycline

Doxycycline can be used once-daily, and therefore has the advantage over oxytetracycline; it is, however, more expensive. The usual dosage is either 50 mg or 100 mg daily. Doxycycline may cause photosensitivity, a problem especially relevant when prescribing for teenagers booked on sunny summer holidays.

Minocycline

Minocycline is a highly effective antibiotic for treating acne. All tetracyclines are lipophilic. There is a lower level of bacterial resistance to minocycline compared with other antibiotics, and there is no cross-reaction in resistance to oxytetracycline and minocycline.

The usual dosage of minocycline is 50 mg twice-daily or 100 mg daily. Minocycline has been used in higher doses in clinical trials, and mega-doses of minocycline (200 mg) daily are used in resistant cases. When prescribed at 200 mg daily, the only dose-related side-effect was pigmentation[16].

There are various forms of pigmentation due to minocycline. Skin pigmentation may be diffuse or localized. The localized form tends to affect scars and the lower legs and may also occur in the mouth and teeth. Minocycline rarely produces urticaria and a photosensitivity rash. The most common colour of pigmentation is blue–black, but a slate–grey purple or brown may also occur (Figure 19).

There have been reports of erythema multiforme, erythema nodosum and Stevens–Johnson syndrome[17]. Minocycline can produce side-effects similar to other tetracyclines, including gastrointestinal problems, vestibular dysfunction, headaches and visual disturbances. Minocycline and other tetracyclines may cause arthritis and arthralgia.

Minocycline rarely causes an eosinophilic pneumonitis. The patient develops dyspnoea, cough and fever and there are radiological signs of pulmonary infiltrates. In these circumstances, the drug has to be withdrawn. Minocycline rarely causes a lupus-like syndrome, which is reversible on cessation of treatment. This treatment has also been associated with an autoimmune hepatitis. Up to 1994, 11 cases of minocycline-induced systemic lupus erythematosus and 16 cases of hepatitis have been reported to the Committee on the Safety of Medicines (CSM). One patient has required a liver transplant and two patients have died[18].

Some healthcare workers have suggested that tetracycline or oxytetracycline should be the first-line treatment of acne[19], because of the higher cost and the rarely reported side-effects of minocycline. Others have recommended that doctors should not change the way they prescribe for acne, and highlighted how uncommon serious complications with minocycline were in their own practices[20]. Since this debate started there has been a decline in the prescribing of minocycline[21]. It would appear that minocycline is a very valuable second-line drug for treating acne.

Lymecycline

This is a tetracycline which has the advantage of a convenient once-daily dosage. It is prescribed as a once-daily 408-mg capsule, which is equivalent to 300 mg of tetracycline base. Lymecycline has been reported to offer similar efficacy to minocycline in the treatment of acne[22] and is less expensive.

Trimethoprim

For many years GPs have used trimethoprim, short-term, to treat acute urine infections, and it has been used long-term for prophylaxis of recurrent renal problems. It is an effective treatment for acne, though it does not have a product license. There is a low level of bacterial resistance. A dosage of 400 mg daily is prescribed, and occasionally higher doses are used. A rash is not an uncommon side-effect, and has been reported in 4% of patients[23]. The drug is well-tolerated, although patients need to be warned of the possibility of a drug rash. Patients do not need regular blood monitoring on this drug. Co-trimoxazole has generally been replaced by trimethoprim.

Antibiotic resistance

Proprionibacterial resistance to both oral and topical antibiotics can develop. Bacterial resistance accounts for approximately 15–20% of failures of treatment in primary care. The concentration of an oral antibiotic in sebum is a factor. Topical antibiotics can reach concentrations which may overcome any resistance. Bacterial resistance is increasing, mostly to erythromycin, less to tetracycline and doxycycline, and the least to minocycline. This increasing resistance is cause for concern. There can be cross-resistance between erythromycin and clindamycin. However, there is no evidence of increased risk of pyogenic infections. In a study of 1000 swabs, *Propionibacterium* acne-resistant strains were found in 25% of samples. Of these, 61% were resistant to erythromycin, 19% to clindamycin and 20% to tetracycline[24]. Interestingly, resistance to minocycline is more of a problem in the USA, and this may reflect the prescribing patterns in different nations.

It is worth considering the possibility of bacterial resistance if the desired clinical response is not obtained. The use of topical antibiotics in combination with benzoyl peroxide or zinc may help prevent the development of resistance. Benzoyl peroxide is equally effective against antibiotic-sensitive and antibiotic-resistant *Propionibacterium* acnes.

To prevent the development of bacterial resistance, patients needing repeat courses should have the same antibiotic. It is better not to use different topical and oral antibiotics in combination, and not to prescribe a topical antibiotic for longer than necessary[22]. During a prolonged course of antibiotics it is worth omitting the antibiotic for 1 week every 6 months and just using topical benzoyl peroxide (this helps to reduce resistant strains of bacteria). Patients with high sebum excretion rates tend to dilute the antibiotic, resulting in poor clinical results. In this situation, megadoses of antibiotics can be helpful. In the UK, oral antibiotics with low levels of bacterial resistance are minocycline and trimethoprim.

Combined oral and topical therapy

Combining an oral antibiotic with a topical therapy improves the response and reduces antibiotic resistance. Ensure the patient understands that these therapies work in different ways, and the

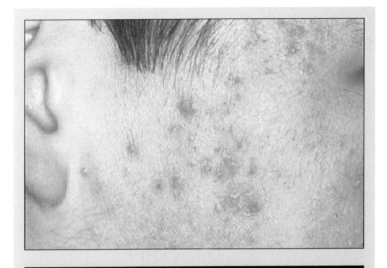

Figure 1. Acne

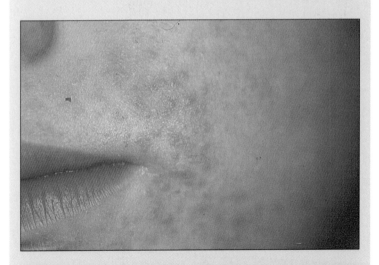

Figure 2. Infantile acne

Figure 3. Acne Scars

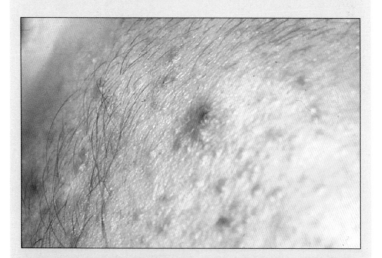

Figure 4. Acne - predominately comedones

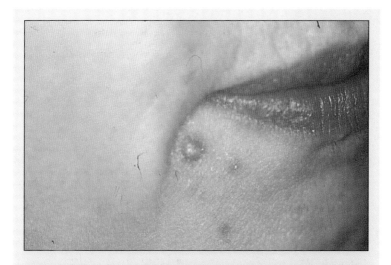

Figure 5. Acne pustule

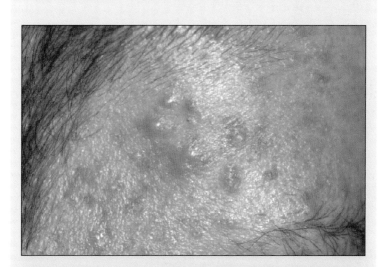

Figure 6. Acne pustules

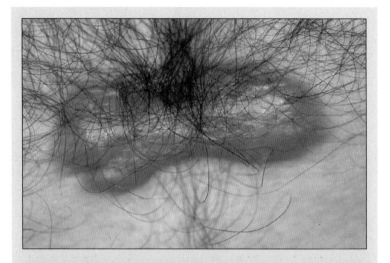

Figure 7. Keloid scar

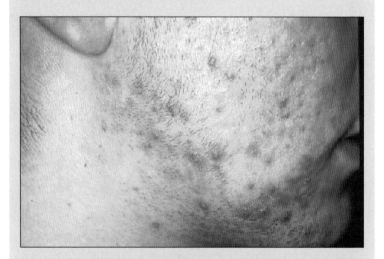

Figure 8. Acne - inflamed lesions

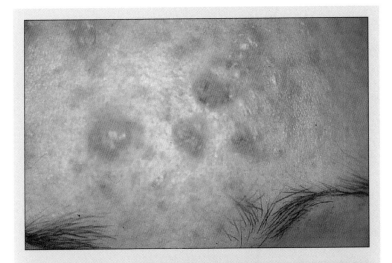

Figure 9. Acne pustules

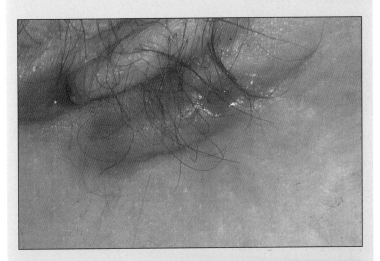

Figure 10. Hydradenitis suppurativa

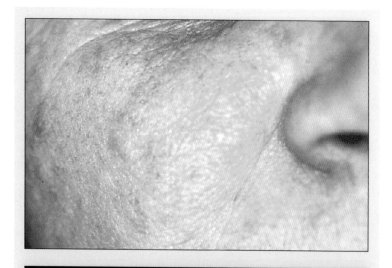

Figure 11. Rosacea

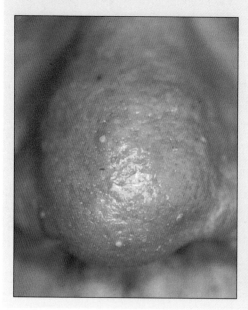

Figure 12.
Rhinophyma/
rosacea

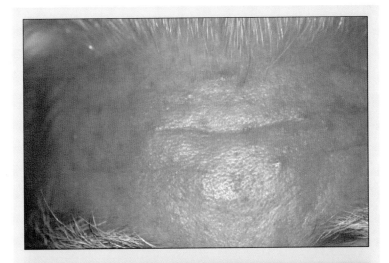

Figure 13. Rosacea

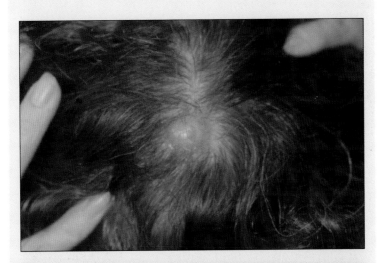

Figure 14. Epidermoid cyst

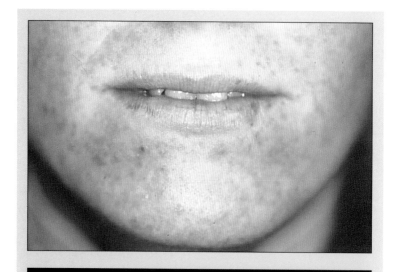

Figure 15. Perioral dermatitis

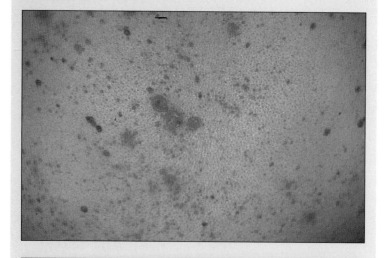

Figure 16. Seborrhoeic dermatitis

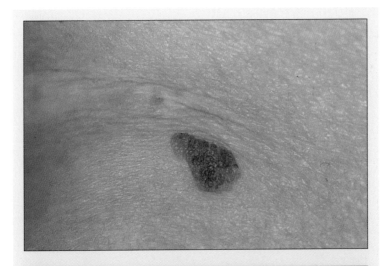

Figure 17. Basal cell papilloma and senile comedone

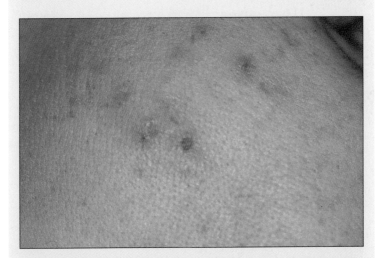

Figure 18. Excoriated acne

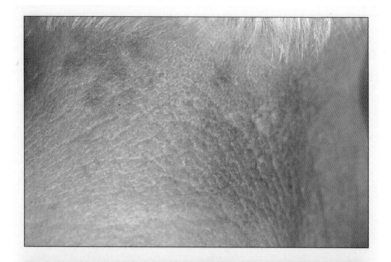

Figure 19. Minocycline pigmentation

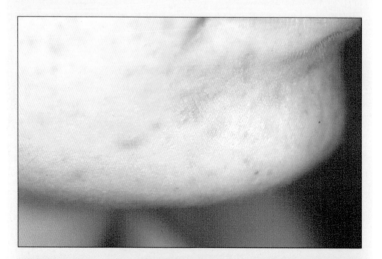

Figure 20. Mild Acne

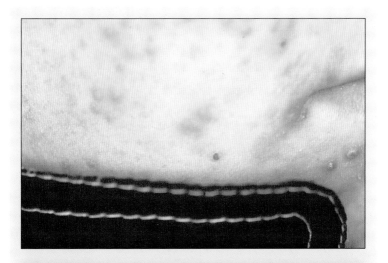

Figure 21. Moderate acne

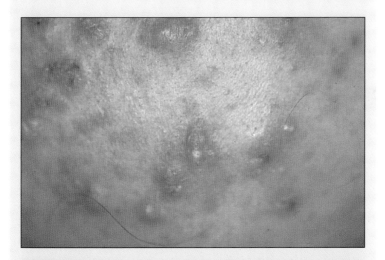

Figure 22. Moderate-severe acne

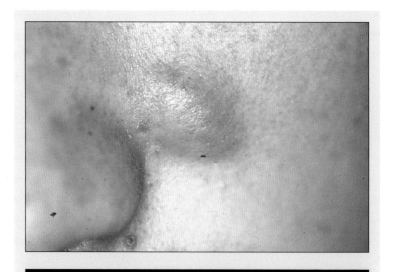

Figure 23. Acne cyst

beneficial effects of taking tablets and applying creams. A simple diagram of the sites of action of different therapies can be useful. Topical retinoids work on comedones and antibiotics work on inflamed lesions. Topical treatments used in combination with oral antibiotics include topical retinoids and benzoyl peroxide.

Chapter Seven

The female patient

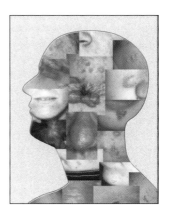

The female with acne

When dealing with patients with acne, females need special consideration. Their acne can be aggravated by certain progesterones and improved with anti-androgens. Potential for interactions between oral antibiotics and oral contraceptives may occur, and certain medications have to be avoided during pregnancy and breastfeeding. Tetracyclines can damage foetal teeth and be taken up into bone.

Hormones and hormonal therapy

Patients prescribed (or athletes self-dosing with) oral steroids may experience an exacerbation of their acne. Progesterones can have androgenic properties. The older progesterones, levonorgestrel and norethisterone fall into this group. The newer progesterones, gestodene and desogestrel are less androgenic, but have been associated with an increased risk of thromboembolism. Norgestimate is a newer progesterone which is less androgenic, and is worth considering for patients with acne. It is available in a combined oral contraceptive. Acne can be improved by reducing the androgenic drive to sebum production and excretion. Possible ways of achieving this include:

1. Displacing the androgens from their receptors

2. Suppression of androgen production

3. Increasing the sex hormone-binding globulin and reducing circulating free androgen

Oestrogens can increase sex-binding globulin and reduce free testosterone. The production of ovarian androgens is reduced when oestrogens inhibit ovulation. Because of their androgenic effect some oral contraceptives can make acne worse. The anti-androgen cyproterone acetate blocks androgen receptors. Spironolactone is another anti-androgen which reduces sebum excretion and may be used to treat acne and hirsutism, although it does not have a product license at the time of writing.

For females with acne, the anti-androgen cyproterone acetate is a possible therapy. Cyproterone acetate may feminize a male foetus, so its use should be avoided during pregnancy. To overcome this possibility it is combined with ethinyloestradiol which has a contraceptive effect similar to that of the combined oral contraceptive pill. Such a treatment may be helpful for those with mild hirsutism and polycystic ovary syndrome. For females who want an acne treatment and need contraception a cyproterone acetate with ethinyloestradiol combination product is very acceptable. A tablet is available containing ethinyloestradiol 35 μg with 2 mg cyproterone acetate. It is considered as appropriate therapy for sexually active females with severe acne who are refractory to prolonged oral antibiotic therapy. The contraindications are the same as any combined pill. GPs should enquire and take note of the patient's age, weight, blood pressure, smoking habits, and family history of thromboembolism. The efficacy of contraception is the same as that of a combined oral contraceptive pill. If the patient does not have a withdrawal bleed after completion of the treatment course, then perform a pregnancy test before continuing therapy. It is theoretically undesirable for a patient to become pregnant whilst on cyproterone acetate, but when this has occurred it has not resulted in any foetal abnormality.

Cyproterone acetate/ethinyloestradiol should be considered for those patients whose acne does not respond to antibiotics, or those who cannot tolerate oral antibiotics. There may be no obvious response for 6 weeks, with improvement occurring during the second or third cycles. The contraindications are the same as for the combined oral contraceptive; nausea, weight gain, and breast tenderness may be caused. Therapy needs to be continued for at least 9–12 months and ensure that concomitant topical therapy is prescribed. Oral antibiotics can interact with cyproterone acetate, so give appropriate advice.

There is no evidence of tachyphylaxis with cyproterone acetate/ethinyloestradiol. When there is not the desired response, i.e. a significant improvement after a reasonable length of time, increase the dose. Extra cyproterone acetate is given, usually 50–100 mg daily, from day 1 to day 10 of the cycle. Cyproterone acetate has a long half-life, and if the increased dose is given for longer in the cycle, it may cause amenorrhoea. Cyproterone acetate/ethinyloestradiol can be given in combination with oral retinoids, in which case establish the patient on cyproterone acetate/ethinyloestradiol before starting the retinoid and continue it after its discontinuation.

Interactions

Oestrogens are absorbed from the small bowel, then metabolized in the liver and excreted in bile. Oestrogens undergo an entero-hepatic circulation, as bacteria in the gut release oestrogen (from oestrogen metabolites) which can then be reabsorbed. Oral antibiotics cause a transient alteration in gut flora and reduces entero-hepatic circulation. Antibiotics may also increase liver degradation of oestrogens.

Patients on the combined pill should take extra contraceptive precautions when starting long-term antibiotics, preferably for 3 weeks. If a course of oral antibiotic impinges on the last 7 days of a packet of pills, then the next course should be started without a 7-day break. It would be reasonable, therefore, to advise the patient not to have the pill-free week if the antibiotic is started within the last 7 days of the current packet. Patients on low-dosage, combined oral contraceptives should have their medication increased from 20-µg to 30-µg pills.

Erythromycin as first choice?

Whilst erythromycin can interact with oral contraceptives, it does not produce the same side-effects in the foetus as tetracyclines. It is worth considering erythromycin as first-line therapy for female patients. However, others believe there is an increasing bacterial resistance to the drug.

The pregnant female

Pregnant females can be treated with oral or topical erythromycin and/or topical benzoyl peroxide. However, other females may become pregnant whilst being prescribed medication. It is therefore advantageous to consider which therapies are contraindicated in pregnancy when prescribing for a female patient. Oral retinoids are highly teratogenic and any female who is going to take these should be aware of this. Topical retinoids are contraindicated in pregnancy, although the risks are probably small.

The GP is in the best position to advise the patient about contraception. Few dermatologists have completed any formal family planning training, and some consider problems beyond the dermis to be outside their realm! The GP is in the unique position of having the medical knowledge and the background information on the patient.

I recommend that all patients on oral retinoids should also be on effective contraception, even if they have not been sexually active. At the end of one clinic, a senior house officer reassured me that contraception was not required as the girl was not married. Thankfully, when I contacted the patient, her education was broader than that of a certain medical school!

Chapter Eight

Oral retinoids

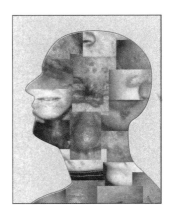

Oral retinoids have revolutionized the treatment of acne. They have a direct effect on the pathological processes involved in the production of acne; sebum production is reduced, as is hyperconification of the pilosebaceous duct. Any associated inflammation is also diminished, as is bacterial colonization. At the present time, the only oral retinoid available for treatment of acne is isotretinoin. Oral retinoids are only available under supervision of a consultant dermatologist, as they are highly teratogenic and expensive. However, they are cost-effective and improve the patient's quality of life.

Indications for oral retinoids

Oral retinoids are indicated for severe nodular acne and severe acne which has not responded to antibiotic therapy. Current practice is to use isotretinoin when the following conditions occur:

1. Severe nodular acne

2. A tendency to scar

3. Dysmorphophobia

4. Severe Gram-negative folliculitis

5. Pyoderma faciale

6. Significant acne which relapses after repeated adequate courses of antibiotic

7. Post-inflammatory pigmentation

It is worth repeating that oral retinoids are teratogenic – a fact that cannot be overstated. This, together with their higher cost are the major factors which limit their usage. It is recommended that oral isotretinoin should be prescribed not only to patients with severe disease, but also to patients with less severe acne, especially if there is scarring and significant psychological stress associated with their disease[25].

The dosage of isotretinoin

The standard dose is 1 mg per kg body weight daily for 16 weeks, although a lower dose of 0.5 mg per kg body weight daily may be used. The lower dose reduces side-effects, but should be continued longer in order to obtain similar results to higher doses. The dosage of 0.5 mg per kg body weight daily can be given for prolonged periods to achieve a satisfactory cumulative dose, whilst reducing the risk of immediate side-effects. Various other dosage regimes have been developed to cover different patient groups, for instance intermittent isotretinoin has been used to treat persistent mild to moderate acne[26]. There may be an initial flare of acne on starting isotretinoin in higher doses. This exacerbation of acne occurs 2–4 weeks after starting treatment and, if it is severe, it can be suppressed by oral prednisolone in a dose of 30 mg daily.

Outcome of retinoids

Within 1 month of commencement, the sebum excretion may reduce by 90%. Expect a 75% cure rate with one 16-week course of oral retinoid. There is a 20% chance of relapse, and if this is the case, then give a second course. Courses of isotretinoin can be continued beyond 16–20 weeks to gain the desired response from those patients who respond slowly.

Advice to patients on oral retinoids

Patients need advice on the benefits and risks of oral retinoids and these should be explained to them carefully. Patient information leaflets are invaluable when patients are considering oral retinoids, however they do not replace face-to-face discussion.

Local side-effects of retinoids

Oral retinoids can produce a variety of side-effects, one of which is dryness of the skin, especially on the face. There may be a mild itch with peeling of the skin. Fissures may develop on the lips which can be treated with emollients. Nose-bleeds can occur; this side-effect may be overcome by applying petroleum jelly. Patients can develop blepharitis and dry eyes; such ocular irritation may require a reduction in retinoid dosage or the addition of a lubricant. In some cases, there may be hair loss and dermatitis (usually facial). Very rarely, hyperpigmentation and sun sensitivity can result.

Possible laboratory abnormalities and screening with oral retinoids

Before commencing oral retinoids, a fasting screen for hypercholesterolaemia and hyperlipidaemia should be performed. Oral retinoids can elevate cholesterol; if cholesterol is significantly elevated at pre-treatment screening, the course of oral retinoid

49

should not be prescribed. Oral retinoids may also raise blood sugar levels in diabetics. Patients with a previous history of gout may suffer attacks. A leukopenia is very rare.

Systemic side-effects

Oral retinoids can cause headaches and, though very rarely, benign raised intracranial pressure. Oral antibiotics should not be prescribed during a course of oral retinoid, as they increase the risk of benign raised intracranial pressure. Oral retinoids may also produce arthralgia and myalgia. There have been reports of a possible link between oral isotretinoin and depression, however this should be placed in context as acne can cause anxiety and depression[27].

Teratogenicity

Because of teratogenicity, oral isotretinoin is a 'hospital only' prescribable drug. Effective contraception is required 4 weeks before and for 4 weeks after cessation of therapy. A pregnancy test is required before commencement of therapy. Retinoids do not affect male or female fertility. Oral retinoids should not be prescribed to breastfeeding mothers. Patients need to be advised not to donate blood during a course of oral retinoid, and for 1 month after its cessation.

Repeated courses of isotretinoin

Some patients need repeated courses of isotretinoin. Very occasionally, patients on long-term oral retinoids develop the DISH (Diffuse Interstitial Skeletal Hyperostosis) syndrome. This can be detected by X-rays of the cervical, thoracic and lumbar spine, knees and ankles, but checks are only required if repeated courses of isotretinoin are needed. Screening should only be considered if patients require multiple courses. Clearly, one has to balance the risks of irradiation against the early detection of side-effects.

Chapter Nine

Protocol for treating acne in primary care

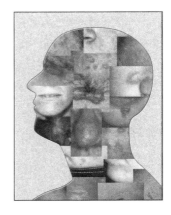

At the initial consultation confirm diagnosis and perform simple grading (Diagram 1). It is important to explore the patient's knowledge of acne, and record any psychological problems related to the acne. Scarring must also be looked for.

Mild acne

Mild acne (Figure 20) can be treated with topical therapy only. Initial treatment is with benzoyl peroxide, and if the desired effect is not obtained at review, adjust the medication (Diagram 2). Comedonal acne responds to topical retinoids/adapalene, whilst inflamed lesions respond to topical antibiotics (Table 2). Adapalene has very good comedolytic activity and anti-inflammatory actions, and is suitable for mild to moderate acne.

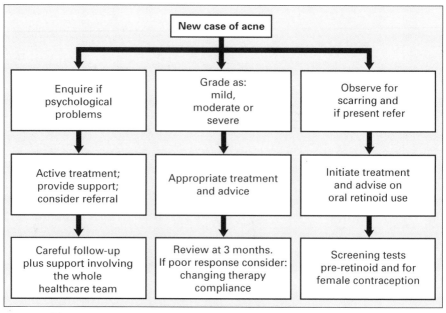

Diagram 1 – Acne action plan: new case of acne

Table 2 – Treatment for mild acne

Type of acne	Treatment
Mild acne	Benzoyl peroxide
Mainly comedonial	Topical retinoids and/or adapalene
Mixed comedones and inflamed lesions	Benzoyl peroxide, adapalene or azelaic acid

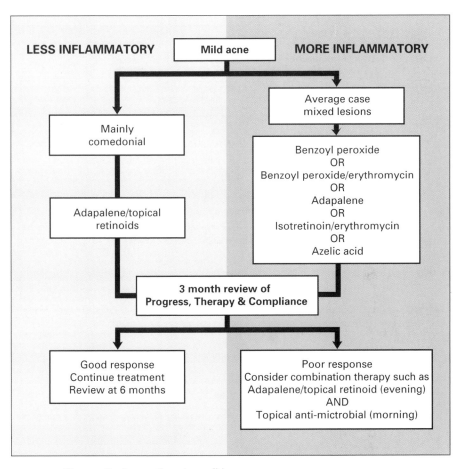

Diagram 2 – Acne action plan: mild acne

Moderate acne

Moderate acne (Figure 21) will require appropriate dual therapy. The usual combination is an oral antibiotic and a topical agent, although there are alternatives (Table 3). Some patients prefer to use topical treatment only, whilst female patients may prefer to take hormonal therapy together with a topical agent (Diagram 3).

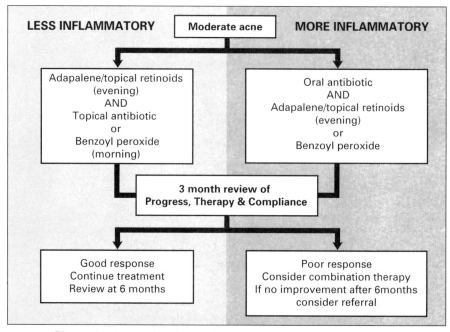

Diagram 3 – Acne action plan: moderate acne

Table 3 – Treatment for moderate acne

Treatment	Topical		Oral
Only topicals	Adapalene/topical retinoid AND topical antibiotic		None
	Adapalene/topical retinoid AND benzoyl peroxide		None
	Topical antibiotic AND benzoyl peroxide		None
Topical/oral	Adapalene/topical retinoid	AND	Oral antibiotic
	Benzoyl peroxide	AND	Oral antibiotic
Alternative for female	Any topical therapy	AND	Cyproterone acetate

Topical agents

A first-line topical therapy would be benzoyl peroxide, but if the patient cannot tolerate it, treatment should be switched to azelaic acid or nicotinamide. Where inflammatory lesions predominate, try a topical antibiotic; where comedones predominate, however, introduce a topical retinoid/adapalene. A combination of topical products is an effective alternative to systemic therapies.

Oral antibiotics

A first-line oral antibiotic treatment is tetracycline or oxytetracycline 1.0 g daily. For females, I often prescribe erythromycin 1.0 g daily (Table 4). Oral antibiotics need to be given in adequate doses and for a reasonable duration. Where compliance is a problem consider lymecycline, doxycycline or minocycline.

Table 4 – Choice of oral antibiotics

Situation	Treatment	Alternatives
Routine	Oxytetracycline	Erythromycin
Female patients	Erythromycin	Oxytetracycline
If possible poor compliance	Lymecycline	Doxycycline, Minocycline
If possible resistance	Minocycline	Trimethoprim

Review

Patients need regular follow-up in order to observe any change in their acne. GPs should advise on side-effects and check compliance. Therapy for acne takes time, and teenagers are often impatient, wanting a rapid improvement. It is possible to give some idea of the probable rate of improvement expected after an average course of treatment as follows:

1. 30% improvement response after 3 months

2. 60% improvement response after 6 months

3. Significant improvement within a year

4. A minority do not respond

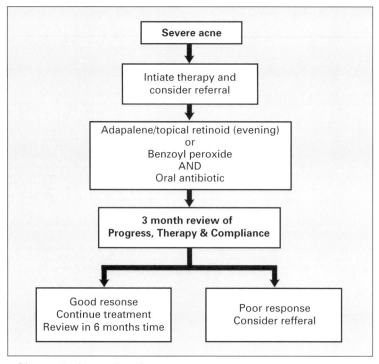

Diagram 4 – Acne action plan: severe acne

Poor compliance or bacterial resistance should be suspected if there is a poor result. At review, check that therapy has been used correctly and was acceptable. If there is no improvement in the acne after 3 months, change the treatment.

Severe acne

Cases of severe acne (Figure 22) should be treated with oral antibiotics and a topical agent, such as benzoyl peroxide, or a topical retinoid/adapalene. If the patient does not respond, then referral is required (Diagram 4). Those patients with nodulocystic and acne conglobata will need immediate referral for consideration of oral isotretinoin. Patients showing a tendency to significant scarring also need referring to secondary care.

Chapter Ten

Audit of acne

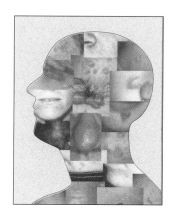

It is possible to perform an audit of a practice's acne care. Review the patient's records for consultations for acne (use of the computer makes this easier). Consider how many patients consulting for acne had a record of:

1. The severity of the condition

2. Presence of scarring

3. Any psychological problems

Also review the following:

1. Treatment

2. Follow-up/outcome

3. Numbers following a protocol

4. Number of referrals

Review the prescribing policy for acne within the practice by considering the following questions:

1. How good is patient compliance?
2. Has the desired course been completed?
3. Is there any system for deciding what is appropriate therapy?
4. Is there some uniformity of advice and prescribing by members of the primary healthcare team?

Chapter Eleven

Physical steps in acne treatment

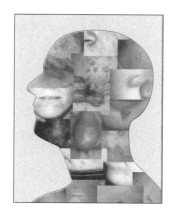

There are five physical steps in acne treatment:

1. Cryotherapy
2. Injection of cysts
3. Phototherapy
4. Treatment of scarring
5. Treatment of comedones

Cryotherapy

Cryotherapy can be used for chronic acne cysts. Two freeze–thaw cycles of 20 seconds are used, the aim being to stimulate polymorphs to the area of the cyst, releasing proteases which destroy the cyst. Cryotherapy can also be used to treat acne keloids, where it has some advantages. Although intralesional triamcinolone is beneficial, cryosurgery is significantly better in early, vascular lesions[28].

Injection of cysts

The injection of triamcinolone into acute cysts (Figure 23) can be helpful. The injection needs to be in the middle of the cyst and care is needed as steroid can cause atrophy if injected into surrounding tissues. No more than 0.25 mg triamcinolone (diluted with sterile saline) should be injected. Whilst injection is effective for acute cysts, cryotherapy is a better treatment for older cysts.

Phototherapy

Light therapy has been used for many years, and acne does improve in the summer with exposure to sun. Visible light has been shown to be a moderately effective alternative for treatment of acne vulgaris[29], but sun-lamp therapy is not as effective as natural light. Superficial X-rays were, at one time, used as a treatment for resistant acne.

Treatment of scarring

Some acne scarring improves with age, although keloids do not. Local atrophic scarring can be treated by collagen injection, but this has to be repeated. Multiple scars can be treated by dermabrasion, but this can produce hypo- and hyperpigmentation, and because of pigmentary changes it is best avoided in the summer. Dermabrasion has been shown to be most effective for treatment of superficial scars, whilst the results of more severe forms of scarring are less predictable[30]. Dermabrasion should only be performed when the acne is under control. Hypertrophic scars respond to intralesional injections and cryotherapy. Laser treatments have been tried for erythematous and hypertrophic acne scarring[31]. Laser resurfacing is effective as a treatment for mild acne scarring, less so in severe atrophic acne scarring[32]. At the time of writing, laser treatment is not generally available through the National Health Service of the UK. Cosmetic camouflage provides a safe mode of help for those with scarring and The Red Cross has made this service available in the UK.

Treatment of comedones

Hot compresses may facilitate the removal of comedones. There are comedone removers which can be used to extract open lesions. Treatment for 2 weeks with topical retinoids/adapalene will facilitate comedone removal. Patients with macrocomedones can be treated with light cautery under local anaesthetic.

Unusual systemic therapies

Oral steroids

Oral steroids, in conjunction with oestrogens, have been used to treat female patients and the resulting decrease in adrenal androgens is beneficial. Oral steroids are given in cases of acne fulminans to suppress the immune response and can also be given with oral retinoids to reduce the initial flare.

Spironolactone

Spironolactone is an aldosterone receptor antagonist which has antiandrogenic effects.

Dapsone

Dapsone is used to treat dermatitis herpetiformis and vasculitis. It can be beneficial in acne, although it needs careful supervision as it can cause a haemolytic anaemia. There is a need to monitor closely the patient's full blood count during therapy. Patients with glucose-6-phosphate dehydrogenase deficiency should not receive dapsone, and some countries screen for this abnormality.

Apppendix I

Self-help

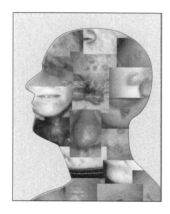

The Acne Support Group provides support, advice and education on acne. They help to dispel myths regarding poor hygiene and diet in the development of acne. In particular, chocolate is falsely incriminated and fried foods do not make acne worse. Acne is not infectious and patients can use cosmetics, although these should be oil-free.

The Acne Support Group
    PO Box 230
    Hayes
    Middlesex
    UB4 9HX

Apppendix II

Formulary

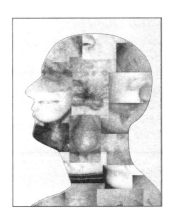

Systemic Treatment

Drug	Dose	Tablets per month	Cost per 28 days (£)	Cost per 84 days (£)
Erythromycin tablets 250 mg	2 BD	112	£12.32	£36.96
Oxytetracycline tablets 250 mg	2 BD	112	£4.36	£13.08
Tetracycline tablets 250 mg	2 BD	112	£3.68	£11.04
Trimethoprim tablets 100 mg	1 BD	56	£1.17	£3.51
Lymecycline 408 mg	1 OD	28	£4.97	£14.91
Minocycline modified release (MR) capsules 100 mg	1 OD	28	£17.62	£52.86
Minocycline tablets 50 mg	1 BD	56	£15.30	£45.90
Doxycycline capsules 50 mg	1 OD	28	£8.06	£24.18

Prices based on drug tariff November 1999

Topical Drugs

Drug	Size	Dose	Cost (£)
Benzoyl peroxide gel	60 g	1–2 times daily	
5%			£3.00
10%			£3.30
Benzoyl peroxide aqua gel	40 g	1–2 times daily	
2.5%			£1.76
5.0%			£1.92
10.0%			£2.07
Benzoyl peroxide gel	40 g	1–2 times daily	
5%			£1.51
10%			£1.69
Benzoyl peroxide cream 5%	40 g	1–2 times daily	£1.51
Benzoyl peroxide lotion	30 ml	1–2 times daily	£1.45

Prices based on MIMS November 1999

Topical Antimicrobial Drugs

Drug	Size	Dose	Cost (£) per 3-month course
Benzoyl peroxide 5%	60 g	1–2 times daily	£9.00
Benzoyl peroxide 5%	23.3 g	Twice-daily	£23.82
Erythromycin 3%	46.6 g	Three months	£45.81
Needs reconstitution		expiry. Store in fridge	
Benzoyl peroxide 5% Potassium hydroxyquinolone sulphate 0.5%	50 g	1–2 times daily	£6.63
Benzoyl peroxide 10% Potassium hydroxyquinolone sulphate 0.5%	50 g	1–2 times daily	£7.47
Azelaic acid 20%	30 g	Twice-daily	£30.00

Prices based on MIMS November 1999

Topical Antibiotics

Drug	Size	Dose	Cost (£) per 3-month course
Clindamycin solution 1%	30 ml	Twice-daily	£13.02
	50 ml		£21.69
Lotion	30 ml		£15.24
	50 ml		£25.41
Erythromycin solution 2%	50 ml	Twice-daily	£25.80
Tetracycline Needs reconstitution	70 ml	Twice-daily Expiry 8 weeks	£18.45
Erythromycin 4% lotion	30 ml	Twice-daily	£21.27
	90 ml	Twice-daily	£61.86
Needs reconstitution		Expiry 5 weeks	
Erythromycin gel 2%	30 g	Twice-daily	£14.91
Erythromycin gel 4%	30 g	Twice-daily	£14.91

Prices based on MIMS November 1999

Duration of treatment with antibiotics: Usual maximum duration 3 months to minimize problems with resistance (course may be repeated after an interval of a few weeks).

Topical Retinoids

Drug	Size	Dose	Cost (£) per 3-month course
Adapalene	30 g	Once-daily at night	£24.00
Tretinoin cream 0.25%	60 g	1–2 times daily	£18.09
Gel 0.01%	60 g		£18.09
Lotion 0.025%	100 ml		£20.82
Isotretinoin gel 0.05%	30 g	1–2 times daily	£19.95
Erythromycin gel 2%	30 g	1–2 times daily	£25.08
Isotretinoin 0.05%			

Prices based on MIMS November 1999

References

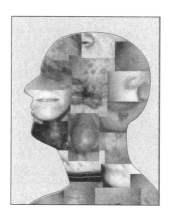

1. Pownall M. Acne Survey. GPs take acne seriously. *Medical Monitor* 20/3/96:65-6.

2. Morbidity Statistics from General Practice Office of Population Census and Surveys 1991-92:54.

3. Rea J. Newhouse M. Halil T. Skin disease in Lambeth: a community study of prevalence and use of medical care. *British Journal of Preventive and Social Medicine* 1976;**30**:107-14.

4. Lello J. Pearl A. Arroll B. Yallop J. Birchall NM. Prevalence of acne vulgaris in Auckland senior high school students. *New Zealand Medical Journal* 1995; **08(1004)**:287-9.

5. Goulden V. Stables G. Cunliffe W. Prevalence of facial acne in adults. *British Journal of Dermatology* 1997;**137** (**Supplement 50**):60.

6. Goulden V. Clark SM. Cunliffe WJ. Post-adolescent acne: a review of clinical features. *British Journal of Dermatology* 1997;**136**(1):66-70.

7. Mills CM. Peters TJ. Finlay AY. Does smoking influence acne? *Clinical and Experimental Dermatology* 1993;**18**(2):100-1.

8. O'Brien TJ. Probable chloracne with the use of a cow udder ointment. *Australasian Journal of Dermatology* 1995;**36**(1):48.

9. Dudley A. Acne Support Group survey results 1996. Personal communication.

10. Cotterill JA. Cunliffe WJ. Suicide in dermatological patients. *British Journal of Dermatology* 1997;**137**:246-50.

11. Motley RJ. Finlay AY. How much disability is caused by acne? *Clinical and Experimental Dermatology* 1989;**14**:194-8.

12. Motley RJ. Finlay AY. Practical use of a disability index in the routine management of acne. *Clinical and Experimental Dermatology* 1992;**17**:1-3.

13. Layton A. Psychological assessment of skin disease. *Interfaces in Dermatology* 1994;**1**:9-11.

14. Cunliffe WJ *et al.* A comparison of the efficacy and tolerability of adapalene 0.1% gel versus tretinoin 0.025% gel in patients with acne vulgaris: a meta-analysis of five randomized trials. *British Journal of Dermatology* 1998:**139 (Suppl. 52)**:48-56.

Grosshans *et al.* Evaluation of clinical efficacy and safety of adapalene 0.1% gel versus tretinoin 0.025% gel in the treatment of acne vulgaris, with particular reference to the onset of action and impact on quality of life. Ibid., 26-33. Shalita A *et al.* A comparison of the efficacy and safety of adapalene gel 0.1% and tretinoin gel 0.025% in the treatment of acne vulgaris: A multicenter trial. *Journal of the American Academy of Dermatology* 1996; **34**: 482-485.

15. Chu AC. Minocycline or oxytetracycline in acne: how should the GP choose? *Pharmacy Dialogue* 1997; **12(1)**.

16. Goulden V. Glass D. Cunliffe WJ. Safety of long term high-dose minocycline in the treatment of acne. *British Journal of Dermatology* 1996;**134:693**-5.

17. Shoji A. Someda Y. Hamada T. Stevens–Johnson syndrome due to minocycline therapy. Letter to *Archives of Dermatology* 1987;**123:18**-20, and Bridges AJ. Graziano FM. Calkoun W. Hyperpigmentation, neutrophilic alveolitis and erythema nodosum resulting from minocycline. *Journal of the American Academy of Dermatology* 1990;**22:959**-62.

18. Gough A. Chapman S. Wagstaff K. Emery P. Elias E. Minocycline induced autoimmune hepatitis and systemic lupus erythematosus-like syndrome. *British Medical Journal* 1996;**312:169**-72.

19. Ferner RE. Moss C. Minocycline for acne. *British Medical Journal* 1996;**312:138**.

20. Cunliffe WJ. Doctors should not change the way they prescribe for acne. *British Medical Journal* 1996;**312:1101**.

21. Ferguson J. Jenkins M. Field J. Letter in BMJ on influence of prescribing minocycline. *British Medical Journal* 1998;**316:** 72-3.

22 Cunliffe WJ *et al*. A comparison of the efficacy and safety of lymecycline and minocycline in patients with moderately severe acne vulgaris. *European Journal of Dermatology* 1998; **8**: 161-6.

23. Goulden V. Aldana O. Cunliffe WJ. Oral trimethoprim - A successful and safe third line acne treatment. *British Journal of Dermatology* 1997;**127**(**Supplement 50**):41.

24. Cunliffe W. Eady A. GP acne survey: results and recommendations. *Prescriber* 19/2/96:87-9.

25. Cunliffe WJ. van de Kerkhof PC. Caputo R. *et al*. Roaccutane treatment guidelines: results of an international survey. *Dermatology* 1997;**194**(**4**):351-7.

26. Goulden V. Clark SM. McGeown C. Cunliffe WJ. Treatment of acne with intermittent isotretinoin. *British Journal of Dermatology* 1997;**137**:106-8.

27. Lamberg L. Acne drug depression warnings highlighted need for expert care. *Journal of the American Academy of Dermatology* 1998;**279**(**14**):1057.

28. Layton AM. Cunliffe WJ. A comparison of intralesional triamcinolone and cryosurgery in the treatment of acne keloids. *British Journal of Dermatology* 1994;**130**(**4**):498-501.

29. Sigurdsson V. Knulst AC. van Weelden H. Phototherapy of acne vulgaris with visible light. *Dermatology* 1997;**194**(**3**):256-60.

30. Aronsson A. Eriksson T. Jacobsson S. Salemark L. Effects of dermabrasion on acne scarring. A review and a study of 25 cases. *Acta Dermato-Venereologica* 1997;**77**(**1**):39-42.

31. Alster TS. McMeekin TO. Improvement of facial acne scars by the 585 nm flashlamp-pumped pulsed dye laser.

Journal of the American Academy of Dermatology 1996;**35**(**1**):79-81.

32. Apfelberg DB. A critical appraisal of high-energy pulsed carbon dioxide laser facial resurfacing for acne scars. *Annals of Plastic Surgery* 1997;**38**(**2**):95-100.

Index

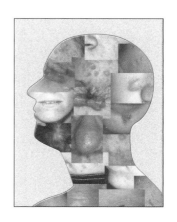

A

Abnormalities, 49

Abnormality, 3, 29, 43, 61

Abscesses, 9, 14

Absesses, 18

Absorption, 34-35

Acne-resistant, 38

Acne, 1, 19, 36, 37, 48

Acnes, 3, 14, 29, 31, 33, 38

Adapalene-like, 30

Adrenal, 61

Afro-caribbean, 12-13

Alcohol, 29

Aldosterone, 61

Allergic, 28

Alopecia, 3

Alveolitis, 73

Amenorrhoea, 43

Amoxycillin, 13

Anaemia, 61

Androgen, 2, 42

Androgenetic, 3

Androgenic, 41-42

Androgens, 2-3, 42, 61

Antacids, 35

Anti-androgen, 42

Anti-androgens, 41

Anti-inflammatory, 4, 28, 30, 33, 51

Antiandrogenic, 61

Antiandrogens, 9
Antibacterial, 28, 32
Antibiotic-resistant, 38
Antibiotic-sensitive, 38
Anticoagulants, 33
Anticomedogenic, 29
Anticomedonal, 28-29
Anticonvulsants, 4
Antifungal, 32
Antimicrobial, 67
Antiseptics, 12
Apsea, 19, 21, 23
Arthralgia, 36, 50
Arthritis, 36
Astemizole, 35
Atrophic, 8-9, 60
Atrophy, 60
Autoimmune, 36, 73
Axillae, 9

B

Bacteria, 3, 38, 44
Barbae, 12
Basal, 12
Beard, 12
Bedding, 28
Benign, 34, 50
Bile, 44
Blackheads, 3, 7
Bleaching, 28
Blepharitis, 10, 49
Boils, 11

Bone, 41
Bones, 34
Bowel, 44
Breast, 43
Breastfeeding, 34, 41, 50

C

Calcium, 35
Camouflage, 61
Candidal, 33
Carbamazepine, 35
Carcinoma, 12
Cautery, 61
Celts, 10
Cervical, 50
Chest, 2, 9, 11, 18
Children, 19, 34
Chins, 4
Chloracne, 72
Chloramphenicol, 29
Chocolate, 63
Cholesterol, 49
Cisapride, 35
Clindamycin, 29, 38, 68
Clonidine, 10
Co-trimoxazole, 37
Coal, 4
Cobblestone, 12
Collagen, 8, 60
Colonization, 4, 47
Colonized, 3
Comedo, 10

Comedolytic, 30, 51
Comedonal, 51
Comedone, 61
Comedonial, 52
Compresses, 61
Concomitant, 43
Conglobata, 14, 56
Conjunctivitis, 10
Contraception, 42-43, 45, 50
Contraceptive, 17, 42-44
Cosmetic, 61
Cosmetics, 4, 63
Cream, 28, 30, 32, 66, 69
Creams, 39
Cruciate, 10
Cryosurgery, 59, 74
Cryotherapy, 59-60
Cyclosporin, 35
Cyst, 59-60
Cytokines, 4

D
Dapsone, 61
Degradation, 44
Dehydrogenase, 61
Demodex, 9
Dermabrasion, 60, 74
Dermatitis, 11, 28, 49, 61
Dermato-venereologica, 74
Dermatophyte, 12
Dermis, 45
Desogestrel, 42

Desquamation, 31
Diabetics, 50
Dihydrotestosterone, 3
Dioxide, 75
Discontinuation, 43
Doxycycline, 33-35, 37, 55, 65
Ducts, 3-4
Dysmorphophobia, 17, 19, 48
Dyspnoea, 36

E
Egyptians, 31
Emollient, 30
Emollients, 28, 49
Employment, 19, 23
Endocrine, 3
Enterohepatic, 44
Eosinophilic, 36
Epidermidis, 3
Epidermoid, 11
Epilepsy, 12
Eruption, 33
Erythema, 10, 14, 36, 73
Erythematosus, 36
Erythematosus-like, 73
Erythematous, 11, 60
Ethinyloestradiol, 42-43, 53
Exacerbation, 41, 48
Excoriated, 29
Excoriee, 13
Excretion, 38, 42, 49
Exercise, 25

Eyelid, 11
Eyes, 49

F

Face, 2, 7, 9-12, 49
Facial, 2, 9-10, 18, 49, 71,
74-75
Faciale, 13, 48
Fair-skinned, 10
Fertility, 50
Fever, 14, 36
Fibrotic, 8
Fissures, 49
Flashlamp-pumped, 74
Flexures, 9
Flora, 44
Fluorescence, 29
Flushing, 10
Follicle, 3
Follicles, 7-8
Follicular, 8, 28
Folliculitis, 11, 13, 48
Freeze–thaw, 59
Fulminans, 13-14, 61
Fungal, 12

G

Gastrointestinal, 33, 36
Genetic, 2
Gestodene, 42
Globulin, 42

Glucose-6-phosphate, 61
Gold, 28
Gout, 50
Grading, 17-18, 25, 51
Gram-negative, 13, 48
Groin, 9

H

Haemolytic, 61
Hair, 7, 28, 49
Halogenated, 5
Headaches, 36, 50
Hepatitis, 36, 73
Herpetiformis, 61
Hirsutism, 42
Hormonal, 3, 41, 52
Hormone-binding, 42
Hormones, 41
Hydrocarbons, 4-5
Hydroxyquinolone, 67
Hyperandrogenicity, 2
Hypercholesterolaemia, 49
Hyperconification, 3, 29, 47
Hyperkeratinization, 8
Hyperlipidaemia, 49
Hyperostosis, 50
Hyperpigmentation, 13, 49,
60, 73
Hyperplastic, 12
Hyperproliferation, 3
Hypertrophic, 8, 60
Hypoand, 60

I

Ice-pick, 8
Imidazoles, 11, 32
Infection, 11-12
Infections, 35, 37-38
Infectious, 63
Inflammation, 12, 47
Inherited, 12
Interstitial, 50
Intracranial, 34, 50
Intralesional, 59-60, 74
Iron, 35
Irradiation, 50
Irritant, 28
Irritation, 28-31, 49

K

Keloid, 8, 10
Keloids, 59-60, 74
Keratinization, 28
Keratolytic, 28, 31

L

Laser, 10, 60, 74-75
Leisions, 18
Leucocytosis, 14
Leukopenia, 50
Levonorgestrel, 41
Lipase, 4
Lipids, 17
Lipophilic, 35

Lithium, 4
Liver, 17, 35-36, 44
Lupus, 36, 73
Lupus-like, 36
Lymecycline, 33-34, 37, 55,
  65, 74
Lymphocyte, 4

M

Macrocomedones, 61
Macular, 9
Macules, 8-9
Majorca, 4
Melanin, 8
Metronidazole, 10
Miconazole, 32
Microcomedones, 3, 29
Minocycline-induced, 36
Minocycline, 37
Myalgia, 50
Mycological, 12

N

Naevi, 12
Naevus, 10
Nasolabial, 11
Nausea, 43
Neck, 4, 10
Necrosis, 10
Neomycin, 29
Neutrophil, 30
Neutrophilic, 73

Nicotinamide, 27, 30, 55
Nicotine, 4
Nodosum, 14, 36, 73
Nodular, 14, 47-48
Nodules, 7-9, 14
Nodulocystic, 17, 56
Norethisterone, 41
Norgestimate, 42

O
Oestrogen, 44
Oestrogens, 42, 44, 61
Oils, 4-5
Ovale, 3
Ovarian, 42
Ovaries, 3
Ovary, 42
Ovulation, 42
Oxytetracyline, 34

P
Pathogen, 13
Pathogens, 13
Periods, 48
Perioral, 11
Petaloid, 11
Petroleum, 49
Photodamage, 9
Photosensitivity, 28, 35-36
Photosensitization, 30
Phototherapy, 59-60, 74
Phototoxicity, 33

Pigmentation, 28, 36, 48
Pigmentation, 35
Pilosebaceous, 3, 8, 12, 29, 47
Pityrosporum, 3, 11
Plaques, 12
Pneumonitis, 36
Polyarthropathy, 14
Polycystic, 3, 42
Polymorph, 4
Polymorphs, 59
Post-adolescent, 2, 72
Post-inflammatory, 13, 28, 48
Potassium, 67
Pregnancy, 28, 30, 35,
    41-45, 50
Premenstrual, 29
Progesterone, 42
Progesterones, 41
Propionibacterium, 3, 14, 29, 31,
    33, 38
Proprionibacterial, 37
Proteases, 59
Proteus, 13
Prurigo, 13
Pruritus, 36
Pseudo-sycosis, 12
Psoriasis, 29
Puberty, 2-3, 18
Pulmonary, 36
Punctum, 11
Pyoderma, 13, 48
Pyogenic, 38

R

Renal, 33, 37
Resurfacing, 60, 75
Retardation, 12
Retiniods, 49
Rhinophyma, 10
Roaccutane, 74
Rosacea, 9-10

S

Salicylic, 27, 31
Scabicide, 31
Scalp, 7, 10-11
Scaly, 11
Scar, 10, 48
Scarring, 60
Sclerosis, 12
Sebaceous, 1-2, 7
Sebaceum, 12
Seborrhoeic, 11, 31
Sebum, 3, 37-38, 42, 47, 49
Smoking, 4, 43, 72
Staphylococcal, 11
Staphylococcus, 3, 12
Steatocystoma, 12
Steroids, 4, 11, 14, 41, 61
Stevens–johnson, 36, 73
Stomach, 34
Suicide, 19, 72
Sulfacetamide, 27
Sulphate, 67

Sulphur, 27, 31
Summer, 35, 60
Sun, 11, 49, 60
Sun-lamp, 60
Sunscreens, 4
Suppuration, 14
Suppurativa, 9, 14
Sycosis, 12
Syndrome, 3, 36, 42, 50, 73
Syndrome, 36

T

Tachyphylaxis, 43
Telangiectasia, 10
Teratogenic, 30, 45, 47-48
Teratogenicity, 50
Terfenadine, 35
Testosterone, 3, 42
Tetracycline, 38
Tetracyclines, 10, 33-36, 44
Thoracic, 50
Thromboembolism, 42-43
Tinea, 12
Topicals, 53-54
Tretinoin, 30, 69, 72-73
Triamcinolone, 59-60, 74
Triglycerides, 3
Trimethoprim, 13, 37-38, 55,
    65, 74
Tuberous, 12
Tumours, 3

V

Vascular, 9, 59
Vasculitis, 14, 61
Vulgaris, 71-74
Vulgaris, 60
Vulvovaginitis, 33

W

Whiteheads, 3, 7-8

Z

Zinc, 29, 31, 38

Abbreviated Prescribing Information for Tetralysal®

Please refer to Summary of Product Characteristics before prescribing.

Presentation: Capsule containing lymecycline BP 408mg (equivalent to 300mg tetracycline base). **Indications:** Acne. **Dosage and administration:** Adults and children over the age of 12 years - One capsule daily for at least 8 weeks. **Contra-indications:** Renal insufficiency. Hypersensitivity. Children under 12 years. Pregnancy and lactation. **Precautions and warnings:** Prolonged use of broad spectrum antibiotics may result in the appearance of resistant organisms and superinfection. Cease treatment if evidence of raised intracranial pressure. Exercise care in hepatic impairment. Tetracyclines may rarely cause photosensitivity. **Interactions:** Antacids and/or iron preparations should not be taken within 2 hours before or after Tetralysal 300. Absorption of Tetralysal 300 is not significantly impaired by moderate amounts of milk. Concurrent use of tetracyclines and oral contraceptives has been associated with a few cases of pregnancy or breakthrough bleeding (not reported for Tetralysal 300). Tetracyclines may enhance the anticoagulant effect of warfarin and phenindione. Co-administration of zinc salts may reduce absorption of both tetracyclines and zinc. **Side effects:** Nausea, vomiting, diarrhoea, erythema (discontinue treatment). Headache and visual disturbances may indicate benign intracranial hypertension. Hepatotoxicity, pancreatitis and antibiotic associated colitis have been reported with tetracyclines. **MA Number:** 10590/0019. **Package quantities and cost:** Calendar pack of 28 capsules £4.97. **Legal category: POM. Full prescribing information is available from the marketing authorisation holder:** Galderma (UK) Limited, Leywood House, Woodside Road, Amersham, Bucks HP6 6AA. Telephone 01494 432606. Fax: 01494 432607. **Date of preparation:** April 1998. **References 1.** Data on file, Galderma.

®denotes registered trademark.

Abbreviated Prescribing Information for EryAcne 2 and EryAcne 4

Please refer to Summary of Product Characteristics before prescribing.

Presentation: Alcohol-based gel containing erythromycin 2% w/w (Eryacne 2) or erythromycin 4% w/w (Eryacne 4). **Indications:** Topical treatment of acne vulgaris. **Dosage and administration:** Apply twice daily. Eryacne 4 is recommended for the first four weeks. If the condition has improved, Eryacne 2 may be substituted. **Contra-indications:** Sensitivity to any ingredient. **Precautions and warnings:** Avoid contact with eyes, nose, mouth and other mucous membranes. Reduce or discontinue use if sensitivity or a severe reaction occur. Cross-resistance could occur with other macrolide antibiotics. **Interactions:** Concurrent topical acne therapy should be used with caution, a cumulative irritant effect could occur. Concurrent use of exfoliants, medicated soaps or cosmetics containing alcohol, a cumulative irritant or drying effect could occur. Erythromycin and clindamycin topical preparations should not be used concurrently. **Side effects:** Dryness, irritation, pruritus, erythema, desquamation, oiliness and burning. Most are related to excipients and are reversible. **Pharmaceutical Precautions:** Store below 25°C. **PL Numbers:** EryAcne 2 PL10590/0021, **EryAcne 4** PL10590/0022. **Package quantities and basic NHS cost:** Tubes of 30g £4.97. **Legal category: POM.** Full prescribing information is available from the product licence holder: Galderma (UK) Limited, Leywood House, Woodside Road, Amersham, Bucks HP6 6AA. Telephone: 01494 432606. Fax: 01494 432607.
Date of preparation: March 1999. (® registered trademark).

Further information is available on request:
Galderma (UK) Limited, Leywood House, Woodside Road, Amersham, Bucks HP6 6AA.
Tel: 01494 432606. Fax: 01494 432607.

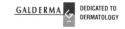

GALDERMA — DEDICATED TO DERMATOLOGY